# ALTERNATIVE CANCER TREATMENT 101

*What You Need to Know About*
*Natural Therapies, Cures and Diets*

# Table of Contents

# Introduction

I want to thank you and congratulate you for downloading the book, "Alternative Cancer Treatments and Recovery: What You Need to Know about Natural Therapies, Cures and Diets".

This book contains proven steps and strategies on how to treat and recover from cancer with the use of natural and safe treatment strategies and diet programs.

This book also contains comprehensive information on alternative cancer treatments in general, its evolution, and its emergence as an effective treatment strategy for cancer patients.

Thanks again for downloading this book, I hope you enjoy it!

# CHAPTER 1

Alternative Cancer Treatments – The Basics

## An Introduction To Cancer

Cancer is defined as the unregulated growth of abnormal cells. Some cancers are localized in a particular part of the body, while others grow and spread into the system.

This lack of a check-and-balance in cell division is usually initiated by a mutation, either by chance, which randomly occurs or is triggered by an environmental factor.

When this happens, cells can reproduce uncontrollably, resulting to a lump in the body.

Among the over a hundred kinds of cancer known to man, approximately 22% has been attributed to tobacco use.

Another 10% compromise of causes associated with obesity, poor diet, sedentary lifestyle and excessive alcohol consumption. The rest of the causes shall be discussed on the latter section.

## Prevalence Of Cancer

In 2012 alone, over fourteen million new cases of cancer were diagnosed. Over 8 million resulted to death.

This comprised approximately 15% of the mortality for that year.

The most common cancers that lead to death are lung cancer, stomach cancer, liver cancer, colorectal cancer and breast cancer.

The following are the most common types of cancer among males: lung cancer, prostate cancer, colorectal cancer and stomach cancer.

On the other hand, the following are the most common types of cancer that affected females: breast cancer, colorectal cancer, lung cancer and cervical cancer. The risk for cancer is proportionally related to age.

Since life expectancy has been increasing, more and more people are now at risk of getting cancer. This is especially true in developed countries, where more people are at risk of being diagnosed with it.

This is perhaps the reason why, despite the advances in oncologic treatment, mortality due to cancer is still increasing.

Although cancer can affect people of different age groups, most of its victims are patients over the age of 65. The incidence of cancer rises with age.

On the other hand, in the United States, around 1 out of 285 children is diagnosed with cancer, with the following kinds as the most common: leukemia, brain tumors and lymphomas.

Despite the increasing trend in the incidence of childhood cancer, mortality in the said age group has been decreasing.

## Causes Of Cancer

As mentioned, a great percentage of cancer cases have been attributed to tobacco use and poor lifestyle choices.

In the developing countries, a huge number has been linked to infections like hepatitis B, hepatitis C and Human Papillomavirus (HPV).

The development of cancer involves interplay of different factors. The following is a list of the possible causes of malignancy:

- Genetics
  - Although cancer may run in the family, it is only in few cases whereby cancer is directly inherited to the offspring. In these cases, genetic testing may be recommended. Usually, gene mutation occurs during a person's lifetime.

- Cigarette-smoking
  - Cigarette smoking has been associated with the development of lung cancer among others.
- Diet and Physical activity
  - Poor eating habits and having a sedentary lifestyle may lead to cancer. In addition, excessive alcohol consumption is also a risk factor for cancer.
- UV exposure
  - Skin cancer has been linked to UV exposure. Among the most common kinds of skin cancer associated with UV exposure are basal cell and squamous cell carcinoma, and melanoma.
- Radiation exposure
  - High doses of x-rays and gamma rays can cause cancer. The atomic bomb survivors in Japan elucidate this. The benefits of radiation exposure for medical purposes should outweigh its costs.
- Other carcinogens

## Benign Vs. Malignant Tumors

There are two basic types of tumors—benign or malignant.

Benign tumors are made up of unregulated growth of normal cells.

Although the cells divide very quickly, they are made up of normal or almost-normal variants. They grow quite slowly and do not spread to other parts of the body.

Benign tumors only become a problem when they grow to a very large size and impinge on other organs, which can become uncomfortable.

Benign tumors can also affect the body negatively when it consumes a huge part of the brain, causing increased intracranial pressure, or when it affects hormonal production and release.

On the other hand, malignant tumors are unregulated growth of abnormal cells. They grow quite quickly and damage the surrounding tissues.

They can also invade through the bloodstream and the lymph, causing the spread of the cancer systemically.

## Cancer Growth And Spread

During the initial growth of cancer cells, they are surrounded with layers of normal tissue. However, during the course of the illness, these abnormal cells penetrate through a barrier known as the basement membrane.

When this happens, the cancer becomes invasive.

The tumor cell is supplied with oxygen and nutrition through a blood vessel. Initially, the blood vessel supplies sufficient amount of oxygen and nutrients for the tumor; but in the end, these become scarce.

As a result, a portion of the tumor dies off.

As a compensating mechanism, the body creates more blood vessels to sustain the needs of the tumor. This occurs in a process known as angiogenesis. Because of this, tumor cell is able to thrive and grow further.

Some anti-cancer drugs actually work against angiogenesis, preventing the growth of tumors.

As the tumor begins to grow bigger, it impinges on its surrounding tissues, applying pressure on them. But eventually, the tumor can spread to the rest of the body.

Three theories can explain this phenomenon:

- Pressure from growing tumor
  - Due to the pressure applied by the growing tumor to its surrounding tissue, it begins to force itself in between the dying normal tissue. Because of this, it is able to go beyond its locality.
- Through enzymes
  - Cells, whether normal or abnormal, all carry with them enzymes that are useful to breakdown themselves during damage. These enzymes are also useful in

wound healing. Tumor cells are thought to possess more of these enzymes to breakdown surrounding normal tissue.

- Through the tissue
  - Scientists have discovered a substance produced by the cancer cells, which allow them to move physically through the normal tissues.

## Signs And Symptoms Of Cancer

During the initial stages of cancer, the patient remains to be asymptomatic. In some cases, patients are diagnosed during the later stages.

This is because of the fact that the symptoms of cancer can mimic those of other conditions. Hence, physicians must be very vigilant in determining signs of malignancy.

The initial signs and symptoms felt by the patient are usually brought about by the local effects of the tumor, depending on where it is situated.

Since cancers are usually composed of mass build-up or ulceration, the initial symptoms may include bleeding or swelling,

As the tumor mestastasizes (spreads to other organs through the lymph nodes and blood vessels), the patient can already feel systemic signs and symptoms like fever, weight loss and fatigue.

## Conventional Drugs Used In The Treatment Of Cancer

Conventional drugs used in the treatment of cancer are classified according to their mode of action, chemical structure and their relationship to other drugs.

The following are the basic classification of conventional chemotherapeutic agents:

- Alkylating agents
  - Alkylating agents act by damaging the DNA and acts in all phases of the cell cycle. Long-term use may

result to damage to the bone marrow. Examples include nitrogen mustards, nitrosureas, alkyl sulfonates, triazines and ethylenimines

- Antimetabolites
  - These drugs interfere with DNA and RNA. They damage the cells during the S phase of the cell cycle. Examples include 5-fluorouracil, 6-mercaptopurine, Capecitabine, Cytarabine, Floxuridine, Gemcitabine, Hydroxyurea, Methotrexate and Pemetrexed.
- Anti-tumor antibiotics
  - Anti-tumor antibiotics damage the DNA of cancer cells. Examples of this are anthracyclin, Actinomycin-D, Bleomycin and, Mitomycin-D and Mitoxantrone
- Topoisomerase inhibitors
  - These drugs destroy the enzyme topoisomerase, which is utilized during the S phase of the cell cycle. They are further subdivided into topoisomerase I inhibitors and topoisomerase II inhibitors.
- Mitotic inhibitors
  - These drugs are derived from plant alkaloids. Although they can damage cells throughout the cycle, they work by stopping mitosis during the M phase.
- Corticosteroids
  - Corticosteroids are hormones and hormone-like drugs, which can be used to treat cancer.

## Common Side Effects Of Chemotherapeutic Agents

Like any other medications, chemotherapeutic are prone to have a number of adverse effects.

The adverse effects and their severity vary among patients. Some patients suffer a lot, while some do not even complain of any.

Some of these side effects may present as symptoms of the cancer itself. Nevertheless, here are the most common adverse effects reported by the patients:

- Fatigue

- o Almost all patients undergoing chemotherapy complain of fatigue. To address this, light exercises and yoga may help.
- Nausea and vomiting
  - o This is also very common among patients. Anti-emetics are usually given to prevent vomiting.
- Hair loss
  - o Hair loss usually begins three weeks after the initial treatment. However, significant hair loss would usually commence around two months later. The hair loss brought about by the medications is temporary. Hair growth resumes after cessation of treatment.
- Increased risk of infection
  - o Chemotherapy puts the patient to an immunocompromised state, which makes them more susceptible to different kinds of infection. To avoid such occurrence, patients are advised to have good hygiene, to do frequent hand washing and to avoid crowded places.
- Anemia
  - o Chemotherapy caused a decrease in red blood cells. Patients usually complain of fatigue and shortness of breath. In worst scenarios, blood transfusion or injection of erythropoietin may be given to the patients.
- Bruising and bleeding
  - o Manifestations of such adverse effect may include bleeding gums, nose bleeding and easy bruisability.
- Mucositis
  - o Chemotherapeutic agents cause inflammation of the mucous membrane lining the digestive tract. It can be felt as pain on the mouth, especially when eating. This symptom is felt approximately a week after the initiation of treatment.
- Loss of appetite
  - o Patients who complain of loss of appetite must be given small frequent meals. If they are not able to ingest food, hospital admission must be considered.
- Effects on skin and nails

- o The skin may become drier, while the nails may become brittle.
- Effects on memory and concentration
  - o Short-term memory loss, concentration and attention span problems may be noted in some patients; however, these will spontaneously resolve after treatment is stopped.
- Sleep problems
  - o Patients usually complain of insomnia, or of waking up in the middle of the night.
- Effects on sexuality and fertility
  - o Some people may lose interest in sex, or may become infertile after chemotherapy. These effects are temporary, but may become permanent in some cases.
- Diarrhea and constipation
  - o Changes in bowel movement may occur after chemotherapy. Other drugs may be given to address these problems.
- Depression
  - o Being diagnosed with cancer can already subject the patient to a certain level of depression. Undergoing chemotherapy aggravates the problem since it makes the patient anxious about his/her condition and the effects of the medications as well.
- Refusal or cessation of treatment
  - o In some cases, patients who are not as responsive to medications, or who are suffering from very severe side effects are no longer compliant to medications. Depression could also play a role in their refusal to take medications.

## Other Treatment Modalities

- Radiation
  - o Makes use of ionizing radiation to target the tumor or to tame the manifestations of cancer. It focuses on the DNA of the cancer cells and spares the normal tissues with the use of shaped radiation beams. This ionizing

radiation is usually in the form of low energy x-rays or high energy x-rays. This kind of treatment is usually used in conjunction with other treatment modalities like surgery or chemotherapy. In particular, radiotherapy is found to be quite effective in cases of painful bone metastasis.

- Surgery
  - This is usually the treatment of choice for cases involving isolated solid tumors. It plays a high role in patients requiring palliative treatment, and has been proven to prolong survival in some cases. In addition, surgery is also a useful tool to establish the diagnosis and as a means for biopsies. In some cases, surgery is all that it takes to make the patient cancer-free.
- Palliative care
  - Palliative care is usually the treatment of choice for patients in whom surgery, radiotherapy and chemotherapy may no longer be useful. It covers other aspects of patient care like emotional, spiritual and psychosocial. The primary goal of this modality is to improve the quality of life of the patient. Although this modality is more useful for patients with later stages of cancer, this should still be provided to all patients for the provision of comfort, especially in the following situations: (1) for people who cannot take care of themselves (2) for patients who did not benefit from conventional treatment (3) and for patients who are deemed to benefit out of palliative care.
- Immunotherapy
  - Although it is still under studies, immunotherapy has been used by some to combat cancer. This acts by improving the patient's immune system, so he/she could withstand the disease.
- Alternative medicine
  - This treatment modality includes a mixture of diverse health care programs, practices and products that are not usually included in conventional medicine. Most parts of this kind of treatment have not yet been proven

by science, but are known by some to be effective; hence it is still continually being marketed.

## Complementary And Alternative Medicine

Alternative cancer treatments are complementary treatments that have not yet been approved by government agencies responsible for the regulation of therapeutic treatments.

These alternative treatments include manual procedures, devices, herbs, chemicals, exercise, and diet.

However, it is important to note that such treatments are not yet supported by studies, either because testing did not result to statistically significant efficacy, or because no proper testing has been conducted.

There were concerns raised concerning the safety of some of these treatments.

There are some types of treatments that were proposed in the past that were found to be unsafe or ineffective based on clinical trials.

However, some of these disproven or obsolete treatments continue to be used, sold, or promoted.

Alternative cancer treatments are often likened to experimental cancer treatment. These methods are still being tested and used experimentally for safety and efficacy.

In addition, complementary treatments may involve non-invasive procedures that are used in conjunction with other treatment.

Traditional chemotherapeutic agents used in treating cancer all went through experimental stages before they were released for widespread use.

Since the 1940s, medical science has developed adjuvant therapy, radiation therapy, chemotherapy, and other newer targeted therapies, including refinement of surgical procedures for the management of cancer.

Prior to the development of such evidence-based modern treatments, about 90 percent of patients with cancer passed away within five years of diagnosis.

With the use of modern mainstream treatments, the number of cancer patients who passed away within the same period was down to 43 percent.

While modern mainstream types of cancer treatment either permanently cure cancer or prolong life, most of these treatments also have adverse effects varying from unpleasant to fatal, including infections, fatigue, blood clots, and pain.

Such adverse effects and the lack of certainty whether the treatment will be successful created a call for alternative treatments for cancer, which was supposed to increase survival rates or cause lesser side effects.

Usually, alternative cancer treatments have not undergone proper and well-designed clinical testing, or the outcomes have not been properly published because of publication biases (refusal to publish research results that are not within the journal's focus area, approach, or guidelines).

Oftentimes, those that were published have very poor methodology. In a recent survey conducted on alternative cancer treatments, it has been reported that almost none conducted dose-ranging studies, which is essential to make sure that patients were provided with a beneficial amount of treatment.

Frequently, such types of treatments appear and vanish.

## Alternative Vs Complementary Treatment

Alternative and complementary cancer treatments are usually clumped together, partly due to the United States Congress'adoption of the phrase "complementary and alternative medicine".

However, experts underscored that the distinction between alternative and complementary therapies is crucial.

Complementary cancer treatments are employed alongside the accepted mainstream treatments.

These treatments tend to be beneficial for the patent and do not involve the use of substances with any pharmacological effects.

These treatments are also relatively inexpensive and are intended for the treatment of side effects rather than to combat cancer cells.

In contrast, alternative cancer treatments are intended to replace the mainstream cancer treatments.

The most commonly used alternative cancer therapies include herbs, nutritional supplements, bioelectromagnetics, mind-body interventions, and restrictive diets.

People who opt for alternative cancer treatments tend to perceive that evidence-based medical treatments are severely ineffective or invasive.

These people are very loyal to their alternative healthcare providers and have a belief that the approach of the treatment must be holistic.

Patients with cancer who opt for alternative or complementary treatments, in conjunction with traditional treatments strongly believe undergoing such procedures gives them a higher chance of survival as opposed to patients who only opt for conventional treatments.

These patients report less depression and anxiety and feel a greater sense of control over their lives.

However, patients with cancer who opt for alternative treatments have a poorer survival time, even after they have taken control of their cancer stage.

About half of healthcare practitioners who dispense alternative or complementary treatments are physicians, although they are usually generalists rather than oncologists.

In fact, for some reasons, as many as 60 percent of physicians in the US have referred their patients to an alternative or complementary practitioner.

## Cam Vs Conventional Treatment

In most countries, conventional and alternative medicine is not usually reimbursable from the healthcare system. Patients need to spend from their pocket to avail of such services.

As opposed to mainstream medicine, whereby licensed specialists are treating patients, providers of CAM usually lack significant training.

Some of them have not even gone through medical school. The protocols used by CAM usually have not gone through thorough research and may have not yet been proven safe and effective.

The lack of conclusions about CAM can be attributed to the scare resources for researches devoted to conventional and alternative medicine.

Lastly, the benefits of CAM may be difficult to quantify, as they are usually intangible and subjective.

## The Need For Complementary And Alternative Treatment

The succeeding chapters contain a list of alternative cancer treatments that have been recommended to prevent or treat cancer in humans.

Most of these treatments however, lack proper medical and scientific evidence in terms of their effectiveness.

Unlike approved cancer treatments, disproven or unproven cancer treatments are usually avoided or ignored by the medical society and are usually considered as pseudoscientific.

Despite this, a lot of these alternative cancer treatments have continued to be promoted as effective, specifically by alternative medicine practitioners. The need for alternative medicine has arisen due to the need to address psychosocial concerns of the patients like stress, anxiety, sleeplessness, and fatigue.

In the United Kingdom alone, 33% of caner patients make use of complementary therapy at some point during the course of their illness. In some kinds of cancer, the number could even go as high as 50%.

According to the Cancer Research (UK), the following reasons make the patient involve complementary and alternative medicine in their treatment process:

- Complementary and Alternative Medicine (CAM) helps make them feel better
- CAM reduced symptoms and side effects
- CAM makes them feel more in control
- CAM makes use of natural and healing therapies
- CAM provides comfort from talk, touch and time
- CAM makes them stay positive
- CAM boosts their immune system
- CAM helps in the search for cures

In general, patients who prefer this kind of treatment find evidence-based medicine as ineffective.

These patients usually pose loyalty to their complementary or alternative medicine practitioners. They gain confidence out of receiving alternative treatments and, possess of greater control of their illness, with less anxiety and depression.

## Safety Of Complementary And Alternative Medicine In Cancer Care

Complementary and alternative medicines are generally safe to use in conjunction with conventional anti-cancer medications.

However, take not that natural does not necessarily mean "safe", and that some may pose some adverse reactions, affecting the mechanism of actions of the former.

An example of this is the influence of antioxidants on the effects of chemotherapy and radiotherapy. Antioxidants are said to protect the cancer cells from the fatal effects of chemo and radiotherapy.

Despite the notions that most patients have on complementary and alternative medicine, their use in combatting malignancy have not yet been thoroughly proven by existing studies.

Hence, it is important to be wary of the possible side effects that these medications may have on the patient.

In addition, the patient must also be aware of the costs of these medications, as they may comprise a significant amount of the total expenses.

As mentioned earlier, CAMs are medications used in dealing with cancer, but their use is proven only as far as testimonials from other patients is concerned.

No studies have guaranteed their use yet, so patients must discuss this with their healthcare team first before involving the said treatment to their anti-cancer therapy.

Some studies have even shown that mortality increases among patients who use complementary and alternative treatment alone.

This numbers are being attributed to the fact that patients with poor prognosis are no longer interested with the said treatments, and patients with good prognosis rely only with the said treatments.

In addition, the time spent on complementary and alternative medicine may hamper the treatment time used for conventional medicine; hence providing ample time for cancer cells to grow.

Complementary treatments that have been found by patients to be helpful when used in unison with conventional treatment include: acupuncture, aromatherapy, massage therapy, meditation, music therapy, spirituality, tai-chi and yoga.

Overall, studies have concluded that complementary medicine can help patients with cancer if they use it with the mainstream treatment.

They are useful in alleviating symptoms of cancer and the side of effects of conventional medications. However, alternative medicines on the other hand, have not yet been proven to have a role in the treatment of cancer.

This goes to show that as far as evidence-based medicine is concerned, alternative treatments still have no role in oncologic treatment.

## Points To Consider Before Engaging In Complementary Medicine

People who are interested to undergo treatment via the complementary method should be aware of the following:

- Inform your physician prior to undergoing any kind of treatment. This may affect the efficacy and efficiency of your medications.
- Determine the goal of the treatment and find out if it will help you.
- Find out all necessary details regarding the treatment, like:
    o Treatment options
    o Risks and benefits of the treatment modalities
    o Treatments, tests and procedures that will be done
    o Difference of the complementary treatment and the standard treatment
    o Your rights to withdraw from the treatment

## Prognosis Of Cancer

The prognosis of cancer depends on the type and the stage at which the cancer has been diagnosed.

Around fifty percent of people diagnosed with the invasive type of cancer die of the disease. In developing countries, mortality is worse due to the types of cancer. In addition, cancer cases in developing countries are diagnosed late.

Despite having survived the disease, cancer survivors are still prone to develop a second type of cancer.

Elderly patients are expected to have poorer prognosis as opposed to patients who are young and healthy.

# CHAPTER 2

## Alternative Cancer Treatments – Synthetic Chemicals and Other Substances

- Vitacor – is a kind of vitamin supplement, which is made popular by Matthias Rath and is heavily promoted online. Vitacor, along with other products under Rath's brand "Cellular Health", are claimed to be effective treatments for cancer as well as other human diseases. Such claims have resulted to Rath's prosecution.

- Urotherapy or Urine Therapy – this treatment involves injecting, drinking, or taking an enema of a person's own urine, or by making or taking some derivative compounds from it, to treat cancer and other types of illnesses.

- Baking Soda or Sodium Bicarbonate – this is a compound with the chemical formula $NaHCO3$ and is at times promoted as cancer treatment by alternative healthcare providers such as Tullio Simoncini.

- Shark cartilage – shark skeleton is grounded and made into dietary supplements and promoted as alternative cancer treatment. This is probably because of the common notion that sharks do not develop cancers.

- Revici's Guided Chemotherapy – a practice that was invented by Emanuel Revici. It involves the use of a chemical mixture, usually composed of various metals and lipid alcohol, which is administered by injection or by mouth. Revici's practice differs from modern chemotherapy despite being named with the same word.

- Quercetin – is a plant pigment that is made into dietary supplements. This pigment is promoted for its ability to treat or prevent cancer.

- Oxygen therapy – an alternative treatment that involves administering oxygen under pressure to bodily openings including the vagina and the rectum. The practice may also involve oxygenating blood or injecting hydrogen peroxide.

- Megavitamin therapy or orthomolecular medicine – a practice that promotes the use of increased doses of vitamins for the treatment of cancer.

- Miracle Mineral Supplement or MMS – is a toxic solution composed of 28 percent sodium chloride prepared in distilled water. This solution is promoted as cure for cancer as well as other types of illnesses.

- Lipoic acid – is a type of antioxidant that is made into a dietary supplement. Its proponents claim that lipoic acid has the ability to slow down the progression of cancer.

- Krebiozen, also popularly known as drug X, substance X, creatine or Carcalon – is a mineral-oil based solution that is promoted as alternative cure for cancer.

- Insulin potentiation therapy – this practice involves the injection of insulin, typically in conjunction with other traditional cancer drugs, with the belief that it will boost the overall effect of the treatment.

- Hydrazine sulfate – also commonly referred to as "rocket fuel treatment"", is a practice that is claimed to treat cancer

- Dimethyl sulfoxide (DMSO) – is a type of organosulfur compound that has been promoted as an alternative cancer treatment since the 1960s.

- Di Bella Therapy – is a practice invented by Luigi di Bella. This method involves the use of a cocktail composed of hormones, drugs, and vitamins and is claimed to be effective in the treatment of cancer.

- Colloidal silver – is a concoction made with a suspension of silver particles that is promoted as an effective treatment for cancer as well as other treatments.

- Khler's autologous tumor therapy or cytokine therapy – this therapy is also sometimes referred to as immunotherapy and involves the use of a therapeutic substrate composed of cytokines. Nikolaus Wlther Klehr, who invented this method, is a dermatologist. He held his private practice in Munich and Salzburg and his patients were mostly from Poanf, Slovenia, and Eastern European countries. Klehr is reported to be claiming that his practice leads to an extended lifespan.

- Chelation therapy – is a practice that involves the elimination of metals from the body through the administration of chelating agents. While chelation therapy is an accepted therapy for heavy metal poisoning, it has also been promoted for the treatment of diseases such as cancer.

- Caesium chloride – is a toxic salt that is promoted as an alternative treatment for cancer on the basis that it has the ability to target cancer cells.

- Cell therapy – is a practice that involves the injection of cellular materials derived from animals in an attempt to treat or prevent cancer.

- Cancell, also called as Entelev, 126-F, JS-101, JS-114, Crocinic Acid, Jim's Juice, Sheridan's Formula and Protocel - is a formula that has been promoted as an alternative treatment for cancer as well as other types of illnesses.

- Apitherapy – is a practice that involves the use of products obtained from bees such as bee venom and honey. Apitherapy has been widely promoted for its anti-cancer benefits.

- Antineoplaston therapy – is an alternative type of chemotherapy promoted in Texas, United States by the Burzynski clinic.

- 714-x – is also commonly called "trimethylbicyclonitramineoheptane chloride, which is a combination of chemicals promoted in the market as a treatment for a wide array of human illnesses including cancer.

# CHAPTER 3

## Plant and Fungus-Based Alternative Cancer Treatments

- Chinese yam or Wild yam — the roots of these types of yams are made into dietary supplements and creams, which are promoted for a number of different medicinal purposes, such as cancer prevention.

- Wheatgrass — is a type of food produced from grains of wheat. Some wheatgrass advocates claim that it can actually shrink cancer tumors.

- Walnuts — referring to the large hard edible seeds of any tree of the genus *Juglans*. Black walnut has been widely promoted as a cancer treatment on the basis that it combats the parasites responsible for the illness.

- Venus flytrap — is a carnivorous herb. The extract of which is used as an alternative treatment for a number of different human illnesses, including skin cancer.

- Cat's claw or *Uncaria tomentosa* — is a woody vine that thrives in the forests of Central and South America. Cat's claw is widely promoted as an alternative remedy for a number of human illnesses including cancer.

- Ukrain — oftentimes referred to as "celadine", Ukrain is a trademarked name of a drug produced from a plant called*Chelidonium majus*. The herbal medication is popularized for its health-giving powers and its supposed ability to cure cancer.

- Graviola or Soursop — promoted widely on the Internet as an alternative cancer treatment.

- Seasilver — is a relatively inexpensive herbal supplement made mostly from herbal extracts.

- *Serenoa repens* or saw palmetto — is a kind of palm tree that thrives in the southeastern United States. The extract of saw palmetto has been promoted as a potent cure for prostate cancer.

- *Trifolium pretense* or red clover — a clover species originating from Europe. This herb is endorsed as a cure for a number of different health conditions, such as cancer.

- Snakeroot or *Rauvolfia serpentine* — an herb used as the basis of natural remedy that some people believe may cure cancer.

- Pau dárco — is a tree found in the rainforest of South America whose bark is oftentimes made into a potent tea. This herbal cure is promoted as an alternative treatment for a wide variety of human illnesses including cancer.

- Noni juice — is a liquid formula derived from the fruit of the tree *Morinda citrifolia*. This tree is indigenous to the Caribbean, Australasia, and Southeast Asia. Noni juice has been recently popularized as an effective cancer treatment.

- Oleander or *Nerium oleander* — is known to be one of the most poisonous commonly planted garden plants. The extract of this poisonous plant is used as an alternative cure for cancer as well as other types of human diseases.

- Mushrooms — are also promoted online as a beneficial cure for cancer.

- Moxibustion — is a practice that is commonly used along with acupressure and acupressure. The practice involves flaming dried-up mugwort leaves close to the patient.

- *Iscador* or mistletoe — is a plant widely used in Anthroposophical medicine. The use of mistletoe as an alternative cancer treatment was proposed by Rudolf Steiner, who believed that the potency of this plant is influenced by planetary alignment when it is harvested.

- Mangosteen – is a kind of fruit found in Southeast Asia and is widely referred to as a "superfruit". The product Xango Juice makes use of mangosteen and is promoted as an effective cure for a number of different human illnesses.

- Juice therapy or juicing – a practice which involves the consumption of juice made with raw vegetables and fruits. This practice has been reported to provide many different benefits including curing cancer and slowing the aging process.

- Chaga mushroom or *Inonotus obliquus* – this is used as a traditional therapy in Siberia and Russia since the 16th century.

- Grapes – is a type of fruit claimed to have anti-cancer effects. The use of grapes as an alternative cancer treatment has been popularized by Johanna Brandt, who invented the "grape diet". Brandt also recently promoted grape seed extract as a powerful cure for different types of illness in humans.

- Gotu kola – a swamp plant thriving in many parts of Africa and Asia. This plant is made into dietary supplements and is promoted as effective alternative treatment for cancer.

- *Hydrastis canadensis* or Goldenseal – is a plant originating from the buttercup family, which is promoted as an effective cure for many illnesses such as cancer.

- Glyconutrients – are kinds of sugars extracted from plants that are primarily marketed under the product name Ämbrotose as an effective alternative treatment for cancer.

- Ginseng – is a type of perennial plant; the root of which is popularized for its many therapeutic benefits, including a claimed ability to combat cancer.

- Ginger – a plant belonging to the *Zingber* family, which is a popular spice in a lot of different cuisine. Ginger is very popular as an alternative cancer treatment for its claimed ability to stop tumor growth.

- Essiac – a mixture of herbal tea invented during the early 20th century and popularized as a form of cancer treatment.

- *Echnicae* – a family of herbaceous flowering plants belonging in the daisy family, promoted as a dietary supplement that can aid in combating cancer.

- Chlorella – a kind of algae claimed to have health-boosting properties, including a claimed ability to cure cancer.

- *Larrea tridentate* or chaparral – an herb used to make a natural cure for cancer.

- Castor oil – a type of oil that is produced from the seeds of the castor oil plant. Claims have been made that the application of castor oil in the skin helps in curing skin cancer.

- Cassava – is a woody shrub that originated from South America. The root of cassava is found to be very abundant with carbohydrates and has been promoted as an effective alternative cure for cancer.

- Carctol – is a type of herbal supplement produced from a number of different ayurvedic herbs. In the United Kingdom, Carctol has been aggressively promoted as an alternative treatment for cancer.

- Capsicum – is a plant belonging to the nightshade family. A wide array of capsicum-based products, including capsules and teas, are made popular for their health values, including as an effective alternative cancer treatment.

- Black salve or Cansema – is a kind of poultice or paste usually marketed as a cure for cancer, particularly skin cancer.

- Cannabis – an herb that is widely used as a medicinal and recreational drug. Chemical compounds produced from cannabis have been widely studied for possible anti-cancer effects.

- Bach flower remedies – are concoctions invented by Edward Bach, in which small amounts of plant compounds are dissolved in a mixture of brandy and water.

- Aveloz, also commonly known as *Euphorbia tirucalli*, pencil tree or firestick plant, which is a succulent shrub found thriving in some parts of South America and Africa. The sap of this plant is used as an alternative treatment for cancer.

- *Andrographis paniculata* – is an ayurvedic medicine herb that is widely made into dietary supplements for cancer prevention and treatment.

- Amygdalin, also commonly known as Laetrile, which is a type of glycoside and is promoted as an effective cure for cancer.

- Aloe – is a type of succulent plant native of Africa. Aloe is also promoted as an effective alternative treatment for cancer.

- Black cohosh or *Actaea racemosa* – is a flowering plant made into dietary supplements. Dietary supplements made from black cohosh are promoted for their health-boosting properties.

# CHAPTER 4

## Diet Based and Alternative Health Systems for Cancer Treatment

Alternative Health Systems

- Naturopathy – is a system of alternative healthcare that is based on a belief in innate energy forces of the body and an avoidance of traditional medicine. Naturopathy is claimed to be an effective alternative treatment for cancer as well as other human illnesses.

- Native American Healing – is a traditional practice employed by some indigenous Americans and which has been promoted to be capable of treating many types of human illnesses, including cancer. This practice of employing community aspects to improve the overall well-being is supported by the American Cancer Society.

- Homeopathy – a pseudoscientific practice of healthcare that uses ultra-diluted compounds. The proponents of homeopathy promote the use of homeopathy as an effective alternative treatment for cancer.

- Holistic medicine – a general term used for the practice of medicine that encompasses spiritual and mental aspects.

- Herbalism – an approach to promote health, wherein potent substances are extracted from the different parts of plants.

- German New Medicine – a popular medical practice popularized by Ryke Geerd Hamer, wherein all illnesses are perceived to be a result of emotional shock. According to this practice, mainstream medicine is viewed as a conspiracy initiated by the Jews.

- Ayurvedic medicine – is a 5,000 year old practice of conventional medicine which traces its roots from the Indian subcontinent.

- Aromatherapy – is a practice that involves the use of fragrant compounds such as essential oils. This practice is based on the belief that smelling fragrant compounds will have a positive effect on one's health. There have been established evidences that show that aromatherapy can actually improve the overall well-being. In particular, it is helpful in relieving pain, nausea and stress.

Diet-based Alternative Treatment for Cancer

- Superfood – a popularized term used to apply to certain types of food with supposed health-enhancing properties. Superfoods are usually promoted as having an ability to cure or prevent diseases in humans such as cancer. Examples of superfood include berries, nuts, green leafy vegetables, citrus fruits, fatty fish, legumes and whole grains.

- Moerman Therapy – devised by Cornelis Moerman, this very restrictive diet is claimed to be an effective alternative treatment for cancer. This diet prohibits the intake of all meats including fish, shellfish, and animal fats. Other restricted food include food coloring, mushrooms, potatoes, cheese, margarine, etc.

- Macrobiotic diet – a very restrictive diet that is based on unrefined foods and grains. This is supplemented by intake of local vegetables. Animal products and highly processed food are also restricted. This diet plan is promoted by its proponents as a means to cure and prevent cancer.

- Kousmine diet – devised by Catherine Kousmine, this very restrictive diet emphasizes grains, vegetables, fruits, pulses, and the use of dietary supplements. This diet plan is claimed to be an effective alternative treatment for cancer.

- Hallelujah diet – is a diet plan is based on the teachings of the bible. This restrictive diet plan focuses on the consumption of raw foods. According to the inventor of this diet plan, it can be an effective alternative treatment for cancer.

- Fasting – not drinking or eating for a certain period of time. Fasting is a practice claimed by some alternative healthcare practitioners to help in combating cancer, probably by starving the cancer tumors.

- Budwig diet or budwig protocol – is an anti-cancer diet that is popularized by Johanna Budwig in the 1950s. The Budwig diet is abundant in flaxseed oil combined with cottage cheese. It also emphasizes meals rich in fiber, vegetables, and fruits. In this diet, meats, salad oil, animal fats, sugars, butter, and particularly margarine are to be avoided.

- Breuss diet – a restrictive diet invented by Rudolf Breuss that is based on tea and vegetable juice. Its inventor claimed that it could cure cancer. The inventory believes that cancer lives in solid food; hence, the tumor will die if the patient will only take vegetable juice and tea for 42 days.

- Alkaline diet – is a restrictive diet invented by Edgar Cayce, which is based on non-acid foods. According to Cayce, his Alkaline diet will have an effect on the body's pH, thereby lessening the risk of cancer and heart diseases.

# CHAPTER 5

## Spiritual and Mental Healing and Physical Procedures as Alternative Treatments for Cancer

Spiritual and Mental Healing as Alternative Cancer Treatment

Below are some alternative cancer treatment strategies that focus on spiritual and mental healing:

- Qigong — the practice of maintaining a state of meditation while making light and fluid bodily movements. This is in the efforts to balance internal life energy. Qigong is believed to have anti-cancer effects.

- Anti-cancer psychotherapy — is a practice that claims that what causes cancer is a "cancer personality". This cancer personality may be treated though talk therapy like that of Deepak Chopra, Bernie Siegel's Exceptional Cancer Patients, and Simonton Cancer Center.

- Psychic surgery — is a trick wherein the practitioner pretends to eliminate a lump of tissue (usually raw animal entrails purchased from a butcher) from a cancer patient.

- Meditation, mindfulness, and transcendental meditation - are mind-body practices wherein cancer patients attempt to master their own mind processes. Meditation, according to the American Cancer Society, may help to improve the quality of life for patients with cancer by relieving anxiety and stress.

- Hypnosis — is a practice that induces a deeply relaxed but alert mental state. There have been claims made by hypnosis practitioners that it can possibly help boost the immune system.

- Faith healing — this practice is said to be a cure to human illnesses by spiritual means, usually by participation in religious rituals and prayers.

- Cancer guided imagery — is a practice that attempts to cure cancer in oneself by imagining it away.

- Music Therapy- a therapy that involves listening to music or playing musical instruments. It may also include writing and composing songs. This kind of therapy is said to control pain, nausea and vomiting.

- Relaxation techniques- a way to calm one's mind and relax the muscles. It may involve visualization exercises and progressive muscle relaxation. This activity is very useful in dealing with anxiety and fatigue and even helps a patient sleep better.

Physical Procedures as Alternative Treatment for Cancer

The following are some physical procedures that are widely used as alternative cancer cures:

- Shiatsu — is a form of alternative medicine that involves the use of massage techniques, stretches, and finger and palm pressure. Shiatsu, according to its advocates, can be an effective alternative cure for many human illnesses, including cancer. In addition, massage can also be a good way to alleviate the pain, anxiety, fatigue and stress experienced by a cancer patient.

- Reiki — is a procedure wherein the Reiki practitioner may look at, blow on, touch, and tap the patient in an effort to influence the energy in their body. Reiki sessions are claimed to be an effective alternative cure for many different human ailments, including cancer. There have been some evidences that show that Reiki sessions are relaxing and may enhance overall well being.

- Dance therapy — is a therapy that focuses on the use of physical movements or dance to enhance physical or mental well-being. Clinical studies indicate that dance therapy may be effective in reducing stress and improving self-esteem.

- Cupping — is a practice where cups are employed to create areas of suction throughout the entire body. Cupping, according to its proponents, can be an effective cure to different types of human ailments, including cancer.

- Colon cleansing — the practice of colon cleansing aims to detoxify the body though the use of enemas and laxatives. In particular, coffee enemas are promoted as an effective therapy for cancer.

- Chiropractic — is a practice that involves the manipulation of the spine to cure a number of different illnesses

- Acupuncture- the practitioner inserts needles into the body. Acupuncture is said to relieve nausea brought about by chemotherapy. In addition, it also alleviates pain.

- Applied kinesiology — the practice of diagnosing and curing diseases by observing and touching the patients to identify significant signs in the muscles.

- Exercise- studies have shown that mild exercise helps relieve symptoms of fatigue and stress and may even help patients sleep better. Exercise is also known to increase lifespan of cancer patients.

- Tai Chi- a form of exercise that merges deep breathing and gentle movement. It is a stress-reliever. However, a patient must see to it that he/she is not bothered or pained by the movements.

- Yoga- is a form of exercise that combines deep breathing with stretching. It is a way by which stress and fatigue are lessened among cancer patients. On top of those, it also provides better sleep.

# CHAPTER 6

# Electromagnetic and Energy-Based and Hybrid Procedures as Alternative Cancer Treatments

Electromagnetic and Energy-Based Alternative Treatments for Cancer

- Zoetron therapy – is a therapeutic practice based around huge electromagnetic equipment that emits a weak field, which is claimed to have the ability to kill cancer cells. In Mexican clinics, patients with cancer who opted to undergo the Zoetron therapy were charged $15,000 for an upfront treatment.

- Therapeutic Touch or TT - is a procedure that does not typically involve touching, opposite to its name. TT is a process wherein the practitioners hold their hands near the patient to impact the inner energy in their body.

- Rife Frequency Generator – a procedure that involves the use of a machine supposed to treat cancer by transmitting radio waves.

- Polarity therapy – is a form of energy medical strategy, which is based on the principle that the negative or positive charge of an individual's electromagnetic field impacts their health. Polarity therapy is promoted as an effective treatment for curing a number of human illnesses, including cancer.

- Orgone – devised by William Reich, orgone is a type of life force that he claims can be gathered to cure illnesses such as cancer.

- Magnetic therapy – the process of putting magnets on and around the body to cure many different ailments. Magnetic therapy has been recently promoted as an effective alternative treatment for cancer.

- Electro Physiological Feedback Xrroid – involves the use of an electronic machine that is promoted to be capable of diagnosing and treating cancer as well as other human diseases.

- Electrohomeopathy, also called as Mattei cancer cure – is a therapy invented by Count Casare Mattei. According to Mattei, the various colors of electricity may be used as a cure for cancer.

- Bioresonance therapy – therapy and diagnosis delivered by connecting electrical equipment to the patient, on the basis that the cancerous cells will emit specific electromagnetic oscillations.

- Hybrid Procedures for Cancer

- Metabolic therapies – is a collective term that refers to enema-and-diet-based detoxification procedures, including the Gerson therapy, which is promoted to treat a wide array of human illnesses, including cancer.

- Lorraine Day's 10 Step Program – a program popularized by Lorraine Day, which is based on behavioral and diet changes, such as ceasing to watch the television or giving up work.

- Livingston-Wheeler Therapy – a therapeutic program that involves a very restrictive diet, the use of enemas, therapy, and various drugs.

- Life blood analysis – this practice involves the testing of blood samples under a high-powered microscope claiming that this can predict and detect cancer and other human illnesses. This will eventually result to a prescription of natural supplements, which are supposed to serve as a form of treatment.

- Kelley treatment – is a program popularized by William Donal Kelley and is based on the Gerson therapy, only with additional features such as osteopathic manipulation and prayers. Steve Macqueen was said to have used this treatment before his death.

- Issels Treatment – a program that is advised to be used in conjunction with conventional treatments. This method requires the elimination of metal fillings from the patient's mouth, and strictly following a restrictive diet.

- Hoxsey therapy – a program that involves the use of an herbal mixture for internal cancers and the use of a caustic herbal paste for external cancers. All these are combined with dietary changes, vitamin supplements, douches, and laxatives.

- Gonzales protocol - a treatment program popularized by Nicholas Gonzales. This program is also based on the Gerson therapy.

- Gerson therapy – primarily a diet program, which limits salt, protein, and other types of food.

# BONUS CHAPTER
## Cancer Prevention

As of present, there is still no guaranteed means to prevent cancer. However, there are some ways to reduce the risk of acquiring it.

Cancer reduction, instead of cancer prevention, focuses on ways by which the risk factors for getting the disease can be diminished. This can be done with the following ways below:

- Early detection
    - The current increase in the prevalence of cancer can also be attributed to the increase in the number of people undergoing screening tests for cancer. Although the prevalence has increased, mortality rates have been decreasing. Early detection leads to early management, which leads to higher chances of survival.
- Eat healthy
    - Cut down on drinks containing high amounts of sugar. Eat more resistant starches as they have been proven to decrease proliferation of rectal tissue. Consuming steamed broccoli also lessens one's chances of acquiring cancer. Brazil nuts, garlic, cauliflower, artichokes, onions, grapes and tomatoes are also notorious for preventing the disease. Drinking one serving of alcohol daily may be protective against cancer. Avoid eating high-fat animal protein. Instead, eat fish or chicken.
- Engage in a healthy lifestyle
    - Studies have shown that individuals who spend most of the day sitting and watching TV have higher chances of acquiring colon and endometrial cancers. Women who exercise are thirty to forty percent less likely to acquire breast cancer.
- Get adequate amount of sunlight
    - According to research, 15 minutes of sun exposure daily is already sufficient to provide the body its

required dose of vitamin D. Adequate levels of vitamin D promotes promote normal cell maturation and reproduction. On the other hand, inadequate levels may lead to certain kinds of cancer, among others.

- Keep your bedroom dark
  - o Ovarian and breast cancer have been associated with increased light exposure at night. Light interferes with the production of melatonin, a hormone responsible for the sleep-wake cycle. A decrease in melatonin promotes estrogen-related cancers.
- Maintain a healthy sexual well-being
  - o Some viruses like the Human Papillovirus (HPV), are sexually transmitted. The said virus is the culprit in causing cervical cancer. It also causes genital warts. Vaccines are now made available.

# BONUS CHAPTER

## Stories of Survivors Who Used Natural Treatments

Although studies have not yet proven the efficacy of alternative medicine as a cure for cancer, these 3 individuals were able to survive the big C without using conventional anticancer treatment.

- Michael Gearin-Tosh
  - He suffered from myeloma (cancer of the bone marrow). He underwent Gerson therapy and acupuncture. He consumed significant amounts of vitamin C and performed Chinese breathing exercises. His doctors gave him less than a year to live, but he was still able to write a book seven years later.
- Yemeni Woman
  - This woman was diagnosed with stage 3 cancer when she was advised to take *Nigella sativa* (black seeds) three times a day with crushed garlic and honey. Three months later, her cancer was reported to disappear.
- Marilyn Brent
  - She is a breast cancer survivor who utilized a diet plan proposed by Solomon J. Wickey, which involves drinking a pint of celery and carrot juice daily, maintaining a healthy diet (no animal protein, peanuts, dairy products, eggs, white flour). She also took some herbs composed of clover blend, apricot extract, food enzymes, parsley and pau d'arco, which she took for 9 weeks.

# Sources:

- Alternative Cancer Treatments: 10 Options to Consider. (2014, December 23). Retrieved from: http://www.mayoclinic.org/diseases-conditions/cancer/in-depth/cancer-treatment/art-20047246

- Chemotherapy Drugs: How They Work. Retrieved from: http://www.cancer.org/treatment/treatmentsandsideeffects/treatmenttypes/chemotherapy/chemotherapyprinciplesanin-depthdiscussionofthetechniquesanditsroleintreatment/chemotherapy-principles-types-of-chemo-drugs

- http://www.cancerresearchuk.org/about-cancer/cancers-in-general/treatment/cancer-drugs/side-effects/what-is-a-side-effect

- http://www.nhs.uk/Conditions/Chemotherapy/Pages/Side-effects.aspx

- http://www.rd.com/slideshows/how-to-prevent-cancer/#slideshow=slide16

- http://www.naturalnews.com/027731_cancer_survivors_natural_remedies.html#

# Conclusion

Thank you again for downloading this book!

I hope this book was able to help you to have a comprehensive understanding on the different alternative treatments for cancer.

The next step is to weigh the pros and cons of each of the presented strategies before deciding to undergo a specific treatment plan.

Finally, if you enjoyed this book, then I'd like to ask you for a favor, would you be kind enough to leave a review for this book on Amazon? It'd be greatly appreciated!

Please leave a review for this book on Amazon!

Thank you and good luck!

www.ingramcontent.com/pod-product-compliance
Lightning Source LLC
Chambersburg PA
CBHW070449290526
45791CB00005B/2102